THE COMPLETE DASH DIET COOKBOOK FOR BEGINNERS

A Complete Budget Friendly, Made Easy Guide To Lowering Blood Pressure With Delicious, Low-Sodium Recipes

BY

Mildred Kent

Copyright Notice

TABLE OF CONTENT

INTRODUCTION

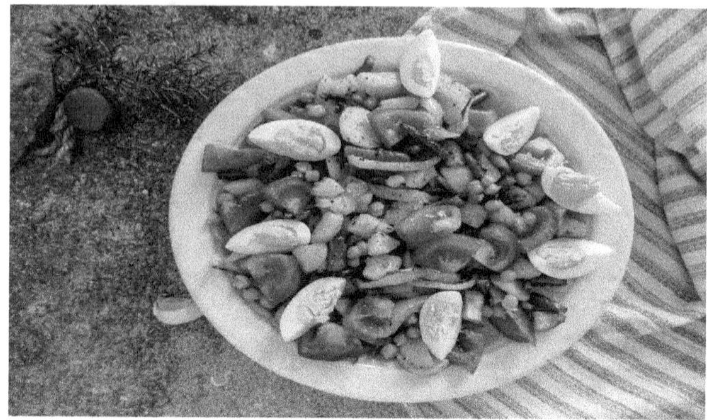

Introduction to DASH Diet Cookbook for Beginners

Welcome to the DASH Diet Cookbook for Beginners! If you're looking to improve your health through better eating habits, you've come to the right place. The DASH diet, which stands for Dietary Approaches to Stop Hypertension, is a well-researched and highly effective way to lower blood pressure, manage weight, and enhance overall wellness.

This cookbook is designed specifically for those new to the DASH diet. We understand that starting a new diet can be overwhelming, so we've made it simple and accessible. Inside, you'll find a collection of delicious and easy-to-follow recipes that adhere to the DASH principles, all aimed at helping you transition smoothly into a healthier lifestyle.

In this book, we cover everything from the basics of the DASH diet to detailed meal plans and practical tips for staying on track. You'll learn about the science behind the diet, the health benefits it offers, and how to set up your kitchen for success. We've also included comprehensive food lists and shopping guides to make your journey as straightforward as possible.

Whether you're seeking to lower your blood pressure, lose weight, or simply eat healthier, this cookbook provides the tools and inspiration you need to succeed. Let's embark on this journey to better health together, one delicious meal at a time!

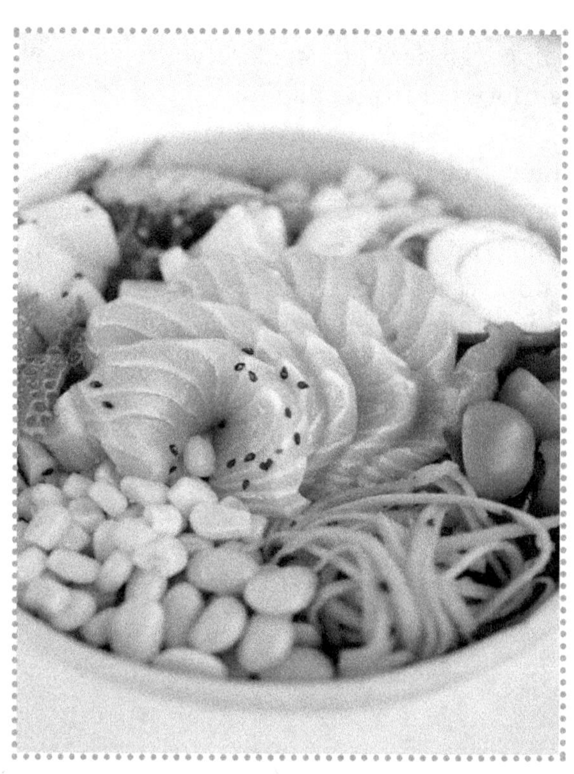

CHAPTER ONE

1. The DASH Diet

The beginning of a healthier, more vibrant you! If you've picked up this book, you're likely looking to make positive changes in your diet and lifestyle. The DASH Diet Cookbook for Beginners is designed to be your friendly guide on this journey, offering you everything you need to start and succeed with the DASH diet.

1.1 Overview of the DASH Diet

The DASH diet, which stands for Dietary Approaches to Stop Hypertension, is a scientifically proven eating plan that focuses on reducing sodium intake and eating a variety of nutrient-rich foods. Developed by the National Institutes of Health, this diet emphasizes the consumption of fruits, vegetables, whole grains, lean proteins, and low-fat dairy, while cutting back on sweets, red meat, and added fats.

This diet isn't about deprivation—it's about making smart, sustainable choices that lead to better health. Whether you're looking to lower your blood pressure, lose weight, or simply eat better, the DASH diet provides a flexible and balanced approach that can fit into any lifestyle.

1.2 Benefits of the DASH Diet

Why choose the DASH diet? Here are some compelling reasons:

1. **Lower Blood Pressure:** The DASH diet is renowned for its ability to reduce blood pressure, which is a major risk factor for heart disease and stroke.

2. **Weight Management:** By focusing on nutrient-dense foods and portion control, the DASH diet can help you shed unwanted pounds in a healthy and sustainable way.

3. **Improved Overall Health:** Beyond heart health, the DASH diet can improve your overall well-being by providing essential nutrients that support bodily functions and protect against chronic diseases.

4. **Simplicity and Flexibility:** Unlike many restrictive diets, the DASH diet is easy to follow and can be adapted to suit your personal tastes and dietary needs.

1.3 Why This Book?

This book is more than just a collection of recipes—it's your comprehensive guide to mastering the DASH diet. Here's why this book is the perfect starting point for your journey:

1. **Beginner-Friendly:** We've crafted this book with beginners in mind, breaking down complex concepts into simple, easy-to-understand information.

2. **Practical Advice:** From meal planning and grocery shopping to cooking tips and dining out, we've got you covered with practical advice that fits into your everyday life.

3. **Delicious Recipes:** You'll find a variety of mouth-watering recipes that prove healthy eating doesn't have to be boring or bland. Each recipe is designed to be nutritious, flavorful, and easy to prepare.

4. **Motivation and Support:** Changing your eating habits can be challenging, but with the right support and motivation, it's absolutely achievable. This book provides you with the tools and encouragement you need to stay on track.

1.4 How to Use This Cookbook

Now that you're excited about the DASH diet, let's talk about how to get the most out of this cookbook.

1.5 Navigating the Book

This book is organized into clear, easy-to-follow sections to help you find exactly what you need:

1 **Part 1:** Understanding the DASH Diet—Learn about the science behind the diet and its benefits.

2 **Part 2:** Recipes—Dive into a variety of recipes for breakfasts, lunches, dinners, snacks, and desserts.

3 **Part 3:** Meal Plans and Shopping Lists—Get started with pre-planned menus and handy shopping lists to make your transition to the DASH diet smooth and straightforward.

4 **Part 4:** Tips and Strategies for Success—Stay motivated and on track with practical tips and strategies.

1.6   Understanding DASH Diet Principles

Before you start cooking, it's important to understand the core principles of the DASH diet. This involves focusing on foods that are rich in potassium, calcium, magnesium, and fiber while limiting sodium intake. These principles are designed to help you maintain a balanced diet that supports overall health.

1.7   Tips for Beginners

Starting a new diet can feel overwhelming, but with these tips, you'll be well on your way to success:

1. **Start Slowly:** Gradually incorporate DASH diet principles into your meals rather than making drastic changes overnight.

2. **Plan Ahead:** Use our meal plans and shopping lists to stay organized and ensure you have all the ingredients you need.

3. **Stay Flexible:** Listen to your body and adjust the diet to fit your personal needs and preferences.

4. **Seek Support:** Don't be afraid to reach out to friends, family, or online communities for support and motivation.

By following the advice and recipes in this book, you're taking a significant step towards better health. Remember, the DASH diet is not a quick fix but a sustainable lifestyle change. Enjoy the journey and the delicious, nutritious food along the way!

CHAPTER TWO

How to Use This Cookbook

Welcome to the second chapter of your journey towards a healthier lifestyle with the DASH diet. This chapter will guide you on how to effectively use this cookbook to get the most out of your DASH diet experience. We'll cover navigating the book, understanding the core principles of the DASH diet, and provide tips for beginners to help you start on the right foot.

2.1 Navigating the Book

To make your experience as seamless as possible, this cookbook is organized into clear, easy-to-follow sections. Here's a quick guide on how to navigate through the book:

1. **Introduction:** The starting point where you'll find an overview of the DASH diet, its benefits, and why this book is your perfect companion.

2. **Part 1: Understanding the DASH Diet:**
This section dives into the science behind the
DASH diet, its history, key principles, and health
benefits. Gaining an understanding of these ideas
will provide you with a strong basis.

3. **Part 2: Recipes:** This is the heart of the
book. It's divided into categories such as Breakfasts,
Lunches, Dinners, Snacks and Appetizers, and
Desserts. Each category offers a variety of recipes
that are both delicious and easy to prepare.

4. **Part 3: Meal Plans and Shopping Lists:**
Here, you'll find 7-day and 14-day meal plans along
with shopping lists to make your transition to the
DASH diet smooth and straightforward. These
plans are designed to take the guesswork out of
meal prep.

5. **Part 4: Tips and Strategies for
Success:** **This section** provides practical advice
on dining out, staying motivated, and overcoming
common challenges.

6. **Appendices:** Includes additional
resources like DASH diet food lists, measurement
conversions, and recommended reading.

The layout is designed to be intuitive, so whether
you're looking for a quick breakfast idea or a
comprehensive meal plan, you'll be able to find it
easily.

2.2   Understanding DASH Diet Principles

Before you dive into the recipes, it's crucial to grasp the core principles of the DASH diet. These principles are the backbone of the diet and understanding them will help you make informed choices.

1. **Reducing Sodium:** One of the main goals of the DASH diet is to lower your sodium intake. This means choosing fresh, unprocessed foods and being mindful of the sodium content in packaged foods.

2. **Increasing Potassium, Magnesium, and Calcium:** These nutrients play a vital role in regulating blood pressure. The DASH diet encourages eating plenty of fruits, vegetables, whole grains, lean proteins, and low-fat dairy to ensure you get enough of these essential nutrients.

3. **Balanced Eating:** The diet is not about extreme restrictions but rather about balance. You'll focus on eating a variety of nutrient-dense foods while limiting sweets, red meats, and added fats.

By following these principles, you'll not only lower your blood pressure but also improve your overall health. Each recipe in this book is designed with these principles in mind, ensuring that your meals are both healthy and tasty.

2.3 Tips for Beginners

Starting a new diet can feel daunting, but with these tips, you'll be well on your way to mastering the DASH diet:

1. **Start Slowly:** Don't feel pressured to overhaul your diet overnight. Begin by incorporating a few DASH-friendly meals into your week and gradually increase from there.

2. **Plan Ahead:** Use the meal plans and shopping lists provided in this book. Planning your meals in advance can save time, reduce stress, and ensure you always have the right ingredients on hand.

3. **Stay Flexible:** Everyone's body is different, so listen to yours. If a particular food

doesn't sit well with you, feel free to substitute it with another DASH-friendly option. The goal is to make the diet work for you, not the other way around.

4.   **Remain Hydrated:** It's critical to consume lots of water. It promotes general health, keeps you full, and aids in digestion. Try to have eight glasses of water or more each day.

5.   **Find Support:** Changing your eating habits is easier when you have support. Share your journey with friends or family, or join online communities of people who are also following the DASH diet. Encouragement and support can have a significant impact.

6.   **Track Your Progress:** Keep a food journal to track what you eat and how you feel. You can do this to recognize trends, maintain accountability, and acknowledge your accomplishments.

Recall that the goal of the DASH diet is to make healthier decisions rather than striving for perfection. One step at a time, and be gentle with yourself if you make mistakes. It matters that you are changing for the better in order to improve your wellbeing.

You will be well-equipped to begin your journey towards a healthier living if you know how to utilize this cookbook, understand the DASH diet's tenets, and pay attention to these introductory guidelines. Cheers to cooking with joy and good health ahead!

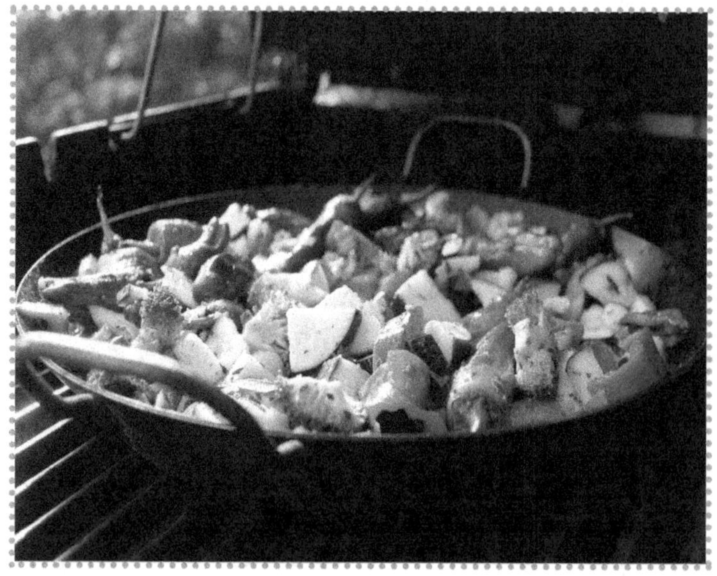

CHAPTER THREE

Understanding the DASH Diet

3.1 The Science Behind the DASH Diet

The DASH diet, which stands for Dietary Approaches to Stop Hypertension, is grounded in scientific research aimed at lowering blood pressure and promoting overall health. The diet was developed through a series of studies sponsored by the National Institutes of Health (NIH). The results were compelling: participants who followed the DASH diet experienced significant reductions in blood pressure, even without reducing their sodium intake. When combined with sodium reduction, the effects were even more pronounced.

The science behind the DASH diet focuses on nutrient-rich foods that are low in sodium and high in key nutrients like potassium, magnesium, and calcium. These nutrients play critical roles in maintaining heart health and regulating blood pressure. By balancing these nutrients, the DASH diet helps reduce the strain on your cardiovascular system, promoting a healthier heart and lower blood pressure.

3.2 History and Development

The DASH diet was first introduced in the early 1990s as a response to rising concerns about hypertension (high blood pressure) and its link to heart disease and stroke. Researchers wanted to find a dietary pattern that could help lower blood pressure naturally, without the need for medication.

The initial DASH study included 459 adults with high blood pressure. Participants were assigned to one of three diets: a typical American diet, a diet rich in fruits and vegetables, or the DASH diet. The DASH diet included fruits, vegetables, whole grains, lean proteins, and low-fat dairy, while limiting red meat, sweets, and saturated fats.

The results were groundbreaking. Those on the DASH diet saw significant reductions in blood pressure within just two weeks. These findings led to widespread recognition of the DASH diet as a powerful tool for combating hypertension and promoting overall health.

3.3 Key Principles

Reducing Sodium, Increasing Potassium, Magnesium, and Calcium

The DASH diet is built around a few key principles that focus on balancing essential nutrients:

1. **Reducing Sodium:** Sodium is known to increase blood pressure by causing the body to retain water, which puts extra pressure on blood vessels. The DASH diet emphasizes lowering sodium intake by avoiding processed foods and choosing fresh, whole foods whenever possible.

2. **Increasing Potassium:** Potassium helps counteract the effects of sodium and reduces tension in the blood vessel walls, which can help lower blood pressure. Foods rich in potassium include bananas, sweet potatoes, beans, and spinach.

3. **Increasing Magnesium:** Magnesium is important for maintaining healthy blood pressure levels. It helps relax blood vessels and supports proper muscle and nerve function. Nuts, seeds, whole grains, and leafy green vegetables are good sources of magnesium.

4. **Increasing Calcium**:** Calcium plays a crucial role in blood pressure regulation and heart health. Low-fat dairy products, fortified plant-based milks, and leafy greens are excellent sources of calcium.

By following these principles, the DASH diet not only helps lower blood pressure but also provides a balanced approach to nutrition that supports overall health.

3.4 Health Benefits

Lowering Blood Pressure, Weight Loss, and Improved Overall Health

The health benefits of the DASH diet extend far beyond just lowering blood pressure. A closer look at what to anticipate is provided here:

1. **Lowering Blood Pressure**:** The primary goal of the DASH diet is to reduce high blood pressure. By focusing on nutrient-rich foods and reducing sodium intake, the diet helps keep your blood pressure in check, reducing the risk of heart disease and stroke.

2. **Weight Loss:** While the DASH diet isn't specifically designed for weight loss, many people find that they naturally lose weight when following it. The emphasis on whole foods, lean proteins, and healthy fats helps you feel full and satisfied, making it easier to manage your weight.

3. **Improved Overall Health:** The DASH diet is rich in vitamins, minerals, and antioxidants that support overall health. By reducing the intake of processed foods and unhealthy fats, the diet helps improve cholesterol levels, reduce inflammation, and boost heart health.

4. **Reduced Risk of Chronic Diseases:** Following the DASH diet can lower your risk of developing chronic diseases such as type 2 diabetes, heart disease, and certain cancers. The diet's focus on whole foods and balanced nutrition provides your body with the nutrients it needs to function optimally.

5. **Enhanced Well-Being:** Many people report feeling more energetic and experiencing improved mental clarity when following the DASH diet. The balanced approach to eating supports not only physical health but also mental and emotional well-being.

Understanding these key aspects of the DASH diet provides a solid foundation for making informed dietary choices. The DASH diet is not just a temporary fix but a sustainable lifestyle change that can lead to long-term health benefits. As you continue your journey with this cookbook, you'll find that incorporating these principles into your daily routine becomes second nature, leading to a healthier, happier you.

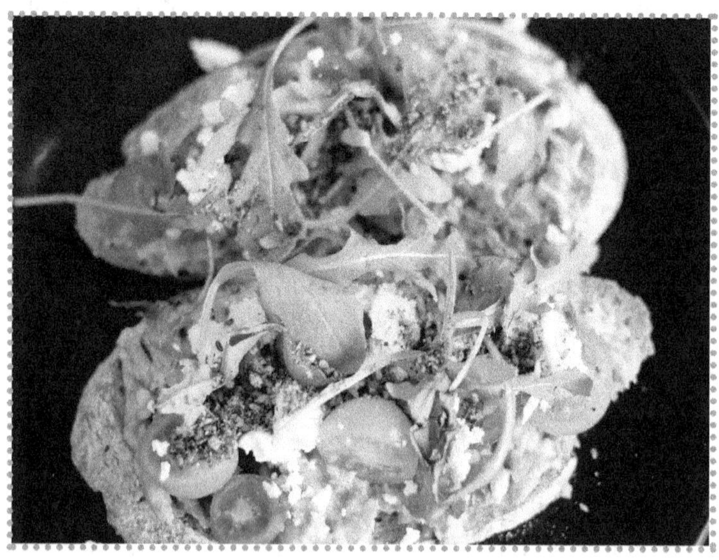

CHAPTER FOUR

DASH Diet Guidelines

4.1 Recommended Food Groups and Serving Sizes

To get the most out of the DASH diet, it's important to understand the recommended food groups and serving sizes. This will help you create balanced meals that provide all the essential nutrients while keeping your sodium intake in check.

1. **Grains:** Aim for 6-8 servings per day. Choose whole grains like whole-wheat bread, brown rice, quinoa, and oatmeal. One serving might be one slice of bread, 1/2 cup of cooked rice, or 1 ounce of dry cereal.

2. **Vegetables:** Eat 4-5 servings per day. Focus on a variety of colorful vegetables such as carrots, broccoli, spinach, and peppers. One serving is typically 1 cup of raw leafy vegetables or 1/2 cup of cooked vegetables.

3. **Fruits:** Consume 4-5 servings per day. Include fresh, frozen, or canned fruits (without added sugar). A serving size might be one medium

fruit, 1/4 cup of dried fruit, or 1/2 cup of fresh, frozen, or canned fruit.

4.   **Dairy:** Aim for 2-3 servings per day. Choose low-fat or fat-free options like milk, yogurt, and cheese. One serving can be 1 cup of milk or yogurt, or 1.5 ounces of cheese.

5. **Lean Proteins:** Have 2 or fewer servings per day. This includes lean meats, poultry, and fish. One serving is about 3 ounces of cooked meat or fish.

6.   **Nuts, Seeds, and Legumes:** Include 4-5 servings per week. Examples are almonds, sunflower seeds, and lentils. A serving size could be 1/3 cup of nuts, 2 tablespoons of seeds, or 1/2 cup of cooked beans or peas.

7.   **Fats and Oils:** Limit to 2-3 servings per day. Opt for healthy fats such as olive oil, avocado, and nuts. One serving might be 1 teaspoon of soft margarine or vegetable oil, or 1 tablespoon of mayonnaise.

8. **Sweets and Added Sugars:** Try to keep these to 5 or fewer servings per week. Choose healthier sweet options and limit sugary treats. One serving can be 1 tablespoon of sugar or jelly, or 1/2 cup of sorbet.

4.2 Foods to Eat and Avoid

To succeed on the DASH diet, it's important to know which foods to include and which to avoid. This will help you make healthier choices and stay on track.

Foods to Eat:

1. **Fruits and Vegetables:** These should be the cornerstone of your diet. They have little calories and a high fiber, vitamin, and mineral content.

2. **Whole Grains:** These provide more nutrients and fiber than refined grains.

3. **Low-Fat Dairy:** Opt for skim or low-fat milk, yogurt, and cheese to reduce saturated fat intake.

4. **Lean Proteins:** Choose fish, poultry, beans, and legumes over red and processed meats.

5. **Healthy Fats:** Use unsaturated fats like those found in olive oil, nuts, and avocados in moderation.

6. **Herbs and Spices**:** Use these to flavor your food instead of salt.

Foods to Avoid:

1. **High-Sodium Foods**:** Avoid canned soups, processed meats, salted snacks, and convenience foods. Check labels for sodium content.

2. **Saturated and Trans Fats**:** Limit butter, fatty meats, full-fat dairy products, and commercially baked goods.

3. **Sugary Beverages and Snacks**:** Reduce intake of soda, candy, and baked goods with added sugars.

4. **Refined Grains**:** Limit white bread, white rice, and pasta made from refined flour.

5. **Alcohol**:** If you drink alcohol, do so in moderation. That's up to one drink per day for women and two for men.

4.3. Reading Nutrition Labels

Learning to read nutrition labels is a crucial skill for following the DASH diet. Labels provide valuable information about the nutritional content of food and can help you make healthier choices.

Key Points to Look For:

1. **Serving Size:** Always check the serving size first. All the information on the label is based on this amount, and it's easy to consume more than one serving.

2. **Calories:** Note the number of calories per serving, especially if you're managing your weight.

3. **Nutrients to Limit:** Aim to keep sodium, saturated fat, trans fat, and added sugars as low as possible. These can contribute to high blood pressure and other health issues.

4. **Sodium:** Look for foods with 5% or less of the daily value per serving.

5. **Saturated and Trans Fats:** These should be limited; try to choose foods with 0 grams trans fat.

6. **Added Sugars:** Less is better. Be mindful of terms like high-fructose corn syrup, cane sugar, and agave nectar.

7. **Nutrients to Get Enough Of:** Fiber, vitamins, and minerals like potassium, calcium, and magnesium are beneficial. Foods with 10% or more of the daily value per serving are considered good sources.

8. **Fiber:** Aim for 25-30 grams per day.

9. **Vitamins and Minerals:** Check for good amounts of vitamins A, C, D, and E, as well as calcium, iron, and potassium.

10. **Ingredients List:** Ingredients are listed by quantity, from highest to lowest amount. Choose products with whole foods listed first and avoid those with added sugars and unhealthy fats near the top.

By mastering these guidelines, you'll be well-equipped to make healthier food choices and fully benefit from the DASH diet. Understanding the recommended food groups and serving sizes, knowing which foods to eat and avoid, and being able to read nutrition labels will set you up for success on your journey to better health.

CHAPTER FIVE

Setting Up Your DASH Diet Kitchen

Welcome to your DASH diet kitchen! Setting up your kitchen properly is a crucial step in making your DASH diet journey smooth and enjoyable. This chapter will guide you through essential tools and equipment, stocking your pantry with staples and fresh ingredients, and effective meal planning and preparation tips.

5.1 Essential Tools and Equipment

To make cooking and meal prep easier and more efficient, it's important to have the right tools and equipment on hand. Here are some essentials for your DASH diet kitchen:

1. **Sharp Knives:** A good set of sharp knives is crucial for chopping vegetables, fruits, and lean meats.

2. **Cutting Boards:** Have multiple cutting boards for different types of food to avoid cross-contamination.

3. **Measuring Cups and Spoons:** Accurate measurements help you stick to the correct serving sizes.

4. **Mixing Bowls:** A set of various-sized mixing bowls is essential for preparing ingredients and mixing salads.

5. **Non-Stick Cookware:** Non-stick pans make cooking with less oil easier and healthier.

6. **Blender or Food Processor:** Great for making smoothies, soups, and sauces.

7. **Slow Cooker or Instant Pot:** Perfect for preparing healthy, home-cooked meals with minimal effort.

8. **Steamer Basket:** Ideal for cooking vegetables while preserving nutrients.

9. **Baking Sheets and Pans:** Necessary for roasting vegetables and baking healthy snacks.

10. **Storage Containers:** Keep leftovers and prepped ingredients fresh and organized.

5.2 Stocking Your Pantry: Staples and Fresh Ingredients

A well-stocked pantry and fridge are key to sticking with the DASH diet. Here's a list of staples and fresh ingredients to keep on hand:

Pantry Staples:

1. **Whole Grains:** Brown rice, quinoa, whole-wheat pasta, oats, and barley.

2. **Legumes:** Canned or dried beans, lentils, chickpeas.

3. **Nuts and Seeds:** Almonds, walnuts, flaxseeds, chia seeds, and sunflower seeds.

4. **Healthy Oils:** Extra virgin olive oil, avocado oil, and canola oil.

5. **Spices and Herbs:** Garlic powder, onion powder, cumin, paprika, turmeric, basil, oregano, and thyme.

6. **Low-Sodium Broth:** For soups and stews.

7. **Vinegars:** Balsamic, apple cider, and red wine vinegar for dressings and marinades.

8. **Canned Tomatoes:** For sauces and soups.

Fresh Ingredients:

1. **Fruits:** Apples, bananas, berries, citrus fruits, and melons.

2. **Vegetables:** Leafy greens, bell peppers, carrots, broccoli, cauliflower, and sweet potatoes.

3. **Lean Proteins:** Skinless chicken breasts, turkey, fish, and tofu.

4. **Dairy:** Low-fat or fat-free milk, yogurt, and cheese.

5. **Eggs:** A versatile source of protein.

6. **Fresh Herbs:** Cilantro, parsley, basil, and mint.

Meal Planning and Preparation Tips

Effective meal planning and preparation can make following the DASH diet easier and more sustainable. Here are some pointers to get you going:

1. **Plan Your Meals:** Take some time each week to plan your meals. Use the meal plans provided in this book as a starting point. Consider your schedule and plan for quick and easy meals on busy days.

2. **Make a Shopping List:** Once you've planned your meals, create a shopping list of the ingredients you'll need. You'll avoid impulsive purchases and save time by doing this.

3. **Prep Ingredients in Advance:** Wash and chop vegetables, cook grains, and portion out snacks ahead of time. It will be simpler to prepare meals during the week as a result.

4. **Cook in Batches:** Prepare large batches of soups, stews, and casseroles that you can portion out and freeze for later. On hectic days, this is a terrific way to save time.

5. **Use Leftovers:** Plan meals that can be easily repurposed into new dishes. For example, use leftover roasted vegetables in a salad or wrap.

6. **Stay Flexible:** Life can be unpredictable, so it's okay to switch things up. Keep some quick and easy options on hand for days when your plans change.

CHAPTER SIX

Breakfasts

There's a good reason why breakfast is frequently referred to as the most significant meal of the day. A nutritious breakfast can set the tone for your entire day, giving you the energy and nutrients you need to stay focused and active. In this chapter, we'll explore a variety of quick and easy morning meals, delicious smoothies and shakes, and whole grain and fiber-rich options to kickstart your day on the DASH diet.

6.1 Quick and Easy Morning Meals

Even though mornings can be hectic, you don't have to forgo breakfast. Here are some quick and easy DASH-friendly breakfast ideas:

1. **Overnight Oats:** Combine rolled oats with low-fat milk or yogurt, chia seeds, and your favorite fruits in a jar. Let it sit in the fridge overnight and enjoy a ready-to-eat, nutritious breakfast in the morning.

2. **Avocado Toast:** Spread mashed avocado on whole-grain toast and top with a sprinkle of salt, pepper, and a dash of red pepper flakes for a quick and satisfying meal.

3. **Greek Yogurt Parfait:** Layer low-fat Greek yogurt with fresh berries, a drizzle of honey, and a sprinkle of granola for a delicious and balanced breakfast.

4. **Egg Muffins:** Whisk eggs with chopped vegetables and pour into a muffin tin. Bake until set, then store in the fridge for an easy grab-and-go option.

5. **Banana Nut Butter Sandwich:** Spread your favorite nut butter on whole-grain bread and add banana slices for a quick and tasty breakfast.

6.2 Smoothies and Shakes

Smoothies and shakes are a fantastic way to pack in a lot of nutrients quickly. Here are some DASH-friendly recipes to try:

1. **Green Smoothie:** Blend spinach, banana, Greek yogurt, almond milk, and a tablespoon of chia seeds for a refreshing and nutrient-packed drink.

2. **Berry Blast:** Combine mixed berries, low-fat milk, a scoop of protein powder, and a handful of oats in a blender for a satisfying and filling smoothie.

3. **Tropical Delight:** Blend mango, pineapple, coconut water, and Greek yogurt for a taste of the tropics in your breakfast.

4. **Peanut Butter Banana Shake:** Mix a banana, a tablespoon of peanut butter, low-fat milk, and a few ice cubes for a creamy and delicious shake.

5. **Avocado Spinach Smoothie:** Blend half an avocado, a handful of spinach, a green apple, and coconut water for a creamy, green smoothie.

6.3   Whole Grains and Fiber-Rich Options

Whole grains and fiber-rich foods are essential components of the DASH diet, helping to keep you full and satisfied throughout the morning. Here are some delicious options to incorporate into your breakfast routine:

1. **Whole Grain Pancakes:** Make pancakes using whole wheat flour or oat flour and top with fresh berries and a drizzle of maple syrup.

2. **Quinoa Breakfast Bowl:** Cook quinoa and top with almond milk, sliced almonds, and dried fruits for a hearty and nutritious breakfast bowl.

3. **Whole Grain Cereal:** Choose a whole grain, low-sugar cereal and top with sliced bananas and low-fat milk for a quick and easy breakfast.

4. **Breakfast Burrito:** Fill a whole grain tortilla with scrambled eggs, black beans, avocado, and salsa for a fiber-rich breakfast.

5. **Chia Seed Pudding:** Mix chia seeds with almond milk and let it sit overnight. Top with fresh fruits and nuts in the morning for a delicious and fiber-packed breakfast.

By incorporating these quick and easy meals, smoothies and shakes, and whole grain and fiber-rich options into your breakfast routine, you'll start your day off on the right foot. The DASH diet offers a variety of delicious and nutritious breakfast ideas to keep you energized and satisfied, making it easier to stick with your healthy eating goals.

CHAPTER SEVEN

Lunches

Lunchtime is an opportunity to refuel your body and keep your energy levels up for the rest of the day. The DASH diet encourages balanced meals rich in vegetables, whole grains, lean proteins, and healthy fats. In this chapter, we'll explore a variety of satisfying salads, hearty soups and stews, and delicious sandwiches and wraps to keep your lunches exciting and nutritious.

7.1 Satisfying Salads

Salads are a fantastic way to incorporate a variety of nutrients into one meal. Here are some DASH-friendly salad ideas:

1. **Greek Salad:** Combine cucumbers, tomatoes, red onions, kalamata olives, and feta cheese. Add oregano, lemon juice, olive oil, salt, and pepper for dressing.

2. **Quinoa and Black Bean Salad:** Mix cooked quinoa with black beans, corn, red bell pepper, cilantro, and avocado. Dress with lime juice, olive oil, and cumin.

3. **Spinach and Strawberry Salad:** Toss fresh spinach with sliced strawberries, walnuts, and goat cheese. Drizzle with a balsamic vinaigrette.

4. **Chicken Caesar Salad:** Use grilled chicken breast, romaine lettuce, cherry tomatoes, and whole grain croutons. Dress with a light Caesar dressing and sprinkle with Parmesan cheese.

5. **Mediterranean Chickpea Salad:** Combine chickpeas, cherry tomatoes, cucumber, red onion, parsley, and feta cheese. Dress with olive oil, lemon juice, and a pinch of salt.

7.2 Hearty Soups and Stews

Soups and stews can be comforting and filling, perfect for a satisfying lunch. Here are some DASH-friendly recipes to try:

1. **Lentil Soup:** Cook lentils with carrots, celery, onions, garlic, and tomatoes in low-sodium

broth. Season with thyme, bay leaves, and a splash of balsamic vinegar.

2.   **Chicken and Vegetable Stew:** Simmer chicken breast with potatoes, carrots, peas, and green beans in a low-sodium chicken broth. Add thyme and rosemary for flavor.

3. **Butternut Squash Soup:** Puree roasted butternut squash with onions, garlic, and low-sodium vegetable broth. Season with nutmeg and a touch of cream.

4. **Minestrone:** Combine kidney beans, zucchini, spinach, tomatoes, and whole wheat pasta in a low-sodium broth. Add Italian herbs for a flavorful soup.

5. **Spicy Black Bean Soup:** Blend black beans with tomatoes, onions, garlic, and cumin. Add a touch of chili powder for heat and garnish with cilantro and lime.

7.3   Delicious Sandwiches and Wraps

Sandwiches and wraps are versatile and convenient for lunch. Here are a few delicious and healthful options:

1.   **Turkey and Avocado Wrap:** Spread hummus on a whole wheat tortilla, add sliced turkey, avocado, lettuce, and tomato. Roll up and enjoy.

2.   **Veggie Wrap:** Fill a whole wheat tortilla with hummus, cucumber, bell peppers, spinach, and shredded carrots. Add a sprinkle of feta cheese.

3.   **Grilled Chicken Sandwich:** Use a whole grain bun, grilled chicken breast, lettuce, tomato, and a smear of avocado.

4.   **Tuna Salad Sandwich:** Mix canned tuna with Greek yogurt, diced celery, and a bit of mustard. Serve with tomato and lettuce on whole grain toast.

5.   **Roast Beef and Arugula Sandwich:** Layer thinly sliced roast beef with arugula, red onion, and a smear of horseradish sauce on whole grain bread.

CHAPTER EIGHT

Dinners

Dinner is the perfect time to unwind and enjoy a balanced and flavorful meal. The DASH diet encourages a variety of lean proteins, wholesome side dishes, and plenty of vegetables. This chapter provides ideas for balanced and flavorful main courses, lean protein options, and delicious sides and vegetables.

8.1   Balanced and Flavorful Main Courses

Main courses on the DASH diet should be both nutritious and delicious. Here are some ideas to inspire your dinner planning:

1.   **Baked Salmon with Lemon and Dill:** Season salmon filets with lemon juice, dill, salt, and pepper. Bake until flaky and serve with a side of steamed vegetables.

2. **Stuffed Bell Peppers:** Fill bell peppers with a mixture of quinoa, black beans, corn, tomatoes, and spices. Bake until peppers are tender.

3. **Chicken Stir-Fry:** Stir-fry chicken breast with a variety of colorful vegetables in a light soy sauce and ginger mixture. Serve over brown rice.

4. **Vegetable Lasagna:** Layer whole wheat lasagna noodles with ricotta cheese, spinach, mushrooms, zucchini, and marinara sauce. Bake until bubbly and golden.

5. **Shrimp and Vegetable Skewers:** Thread shrimp and assorted vegetables onto skewers, brush with olive oil and herbs, and grill until cooked through.

8.2 Lean Proteins: Chicken, Fish, and Vegetarian Options

Lean proteins are a cornerstone of the DASH diet. Here are some options to include in your dinners:

1. **Grilled Chicken:** Marinate chicken breasts in olive oil, lemon juice, garlic, and herbs. Serve over roasted vegetables on the side after grilling until done.

2. **Baked Cod**:** Season cod filets with olive oil, lemon, and thyme. Bake until flaky and serve with a side of steamed green beans.

3. **Lentil Curry**:** Cook lentils with tomatoes, onions, garlic, ginger, and curry spices. Serve over brown rice or with whole wheat naan.

4. **Stuffed Portobello Mushrooms**:** Fill large mushroom caps with a mixture of quinoa, spinach, and feta cheese. Bake until tender and golden.

5. **Tofu Stir-Fry**:** Stir-fry cubed tofu with broccoli, bell peppers, and snap peas in a soy sauce and ginger mixture. Serve over brown rice.

8.3 Sides and Vegetables

Sides and vegetables add variety and nutrition to your dinner plate. Here are some DASH-friendly ideas:

1. **Roasted Brussels Sprouts**:** Toss Brussels sprouts with olive oil, salt, and pepper. Roast until crispy and golden.

2. **Sweet Potato Fries:** Cut sweet potatoes into wedges, toss with olive oil and spices, and bake until crispy.

3. **Garlic Green Beans:** Sauté green beans with garlic and a splash of lemon juice for a simple and tasty side.

4. **Quinoa Pilaf:** Cook quinoa with low-sodium vegetable broth, diced onions, and bell peppers. Fluff with a fork and serve.

5. **Cauliflower Mash:** Steam cauliflower florets until tender, then mash with a bit of low-fat milk and garlic for a creamy side dish.

By incorporating these satisfying salads, hearty soups and stews, and delicious sandwiches and wraps into your lunch routine, and balancing your dinners with flavorful main courses, lean proteins, and nutritious sides, you'll stay on track with the DASH diet while enjoying a variety of delicious meals. Each meal is an opportunity to nourish your body and enjoy the benefits of the DASH diet.

CHAPTER NINE

Snacks and Appetizers

Snacks and appetizers can be part of a healthy diet, especially when they're as nutritious as they are delicious. This chapter provides ideas for healthy snacking, finger foods for gatherings, and tasty dips and spreads that align with the DASH diet principles.

9.1 Healthy Snacking Ideas

Snacking doesn't have to mean reaching for junk food. Here are some healthy snacking ideas that are both satisfying and nutritious:

1. **Fresh Fruit:** Keep a variety of fresh fruits on hand for a quick and natural sweet snack. Berries, citrus fruits, bananas, and apples are all great options.

2. **Nuts and Seeds:** A small handful of almonds, walnuts, or sunflower seeds provides a good source of healthy fats and protein.

3. **Veggie Sticks and Hummus:** Carrot sticks, celery, bell peppers, and cucumbers paired with hummus make for a crunchy, flavorful snack.

4. **Greek Yogurt:** Opt for low-fat or fat-free Greek yogurt. For sweetness, mix with some fresh fruit or a little honey drizzled over.

5. **Whole Grain Crackers and Cheese:** Choose whole grain crackers and pair them with a small serving of low-fat cheese.

6. **Popcorn:** Air-popped popcorn is a whole grain snack that's low in calories. Skip the butter and season with a sprinkle of nutritional yeast or spices.

9.2 Finger Foods for Gatherings

Hosting a gathering or attending a potluck? Here are some DASH-friendly finger foods that are sure to be a hit:

1. **Stuffed Mini Peppers:** Fill mini bell peppers with a mixture of quinoa, black beans, corn, and avocado. They're tasty, colorful, and simple to eat.

2. **Turkey and Cucumber Roll-Ups:** Roll slices of turkey around cucumber sticks and secure with toothpicks for a simple, protein-packed snack.

3. **Caprese Skewers:** Thread cherry tomatoes, fresh basil leaves, and mozzarella balls onto skewers. Drizzle with balsamic glaze before serving.

4. **Whole Wheat Pita Chips and Guacamole:** Make your own pita chips by baking whole wheat pita bread until crispy. Serve with homemade guacamole.

5. **Shrimp Cocktail:** Serve chilled shrimp with a tangy, low-sodium cocktail sauce for a refreshing and elegant appetizer.

6. **Fruit and Cheese Platter:** Arrange a variety of fresh fruits and low-fat cheeses on a platter for a beautiful and delicious snack.

9.3 Dips and Spreads

Dips and spreads can elevate your snacks and appetizers, making them more exciting and flavorful. Here are some healthy options:

1.   **Classic Hummus:** Blend chickpeas, tahini, lemon juice, garlic, and olive oil for a creamy and nutritious dip.

2.   **Greek Yogurt Tzatziki:** Mix Greek yogurt with grated cucumber, garlic, lemon juice, and fresh dill. Ideal for spreading on wraps or dipping vegetables in.

3.   **Bean Dip:** Puree white beans or black beans with olive oil, lemon juice, garlic, and spices for a tasty bean dip.

4.   **Avocado Salsa:** Combine diced avocado, tomatoes, red onion, cilantro, and lime juice for a fresh and zesty salsa.

5.   **Roasted Red Pepper Dip:** Blend roasted red peppers with almonds, garlic, and olive oil for a smoky and flavorful spread.

6. **Baba Ganoush:** Roast eggplant and blend with tahini, garlic, lemon juice, and olive oil for a delicious Middle Eastern dip.

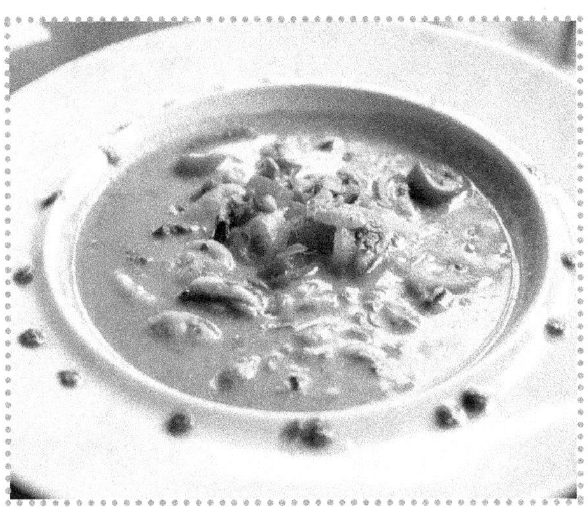

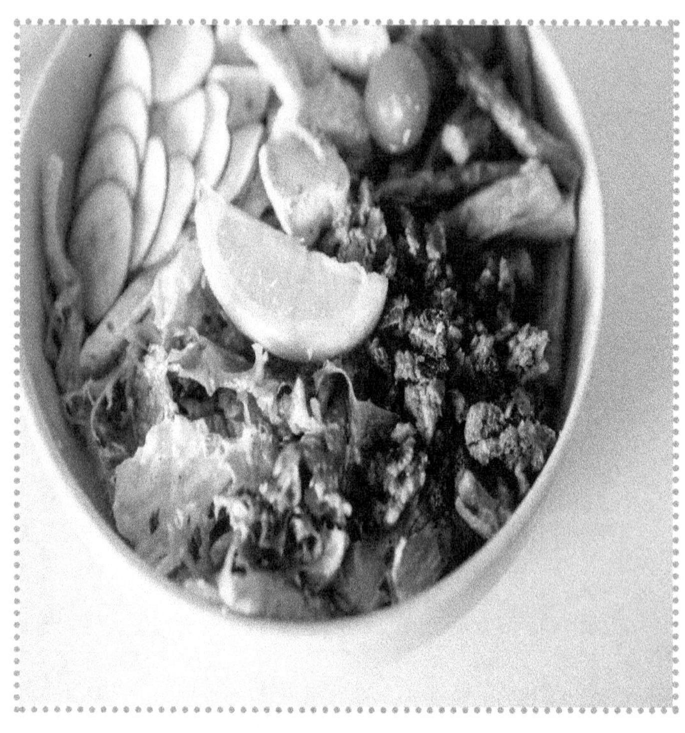

CHAPTER TEN

Desserts

Who says you have to give up dessert on the DASH diet? With a focus on natural sweetness and healthier ingredients, you can enjoy sweet treats that satisfy your cravings without compromising your health goals. This chapter explores sweet treats with a healthy twist, fruit-based desserts, and light and refreshing options.

10.1 Sweet Treats with a Healthy Twist

Indulge your sweet tooth with these healthier versions of classic desserts:

1. **Chocolate Avocado Mousse:** Blend ripe avocados with cocoa powder, honey, and a splash of vanilla extract for a creamy, chocolatey treat.

2. **Oatmeal Cookies:** Make cookies with whole grain oats, mashed banana, and a handful of dark chocolate chips or dried fruit.

3. **Chia Seed Pudding:** Mix chia seeds with almond milk and a touch of honey. Let it sit overnight and top with fresh fruit and nuts in the morning.

4. **Greek Yogurt Bark:** Spread Greek yogurt on a baking sheet, sprinkle with fresh berries and a drizzle of honey, and freeze until set. Break into pieces for a refreshing treat.

5. **Baked Apples:** Core apples and stuff with a mixture of oats, nuts, and a bit of honey or maple syrup. Bake until tender and serve warm.

10.2 Fruit-Based Desserts

Fruit-based desserts are naturally sweet and full of vitamins and antioxidants. Here are some delightful options:

1. **Grilled Pineapple:** Grill pineapple slices and sprinkle with a pinch of cinnamon for a warm, caramelized dessert.

2. **Berry Parfait:** Layer Greek yogurt with mixed berries and a sprinkle of granola for a simple and satisfying dessert.

3. **Frozen Banana Bites**:** Dip banana slices in dark chocolate and freeze for a delicious, bite-sized treat.

4. **Mango Sorbet**:** Puree fresh mango with a bit of lime juice and freeze for a refreshing, homemade sorbet.

4. **Fruit Salad**:** Mix a variety of your favorite fruits with a squeeze of lime juice and a handful of fresh mint leaves for a vibrant fruit salad.

6. **Poached Pears**:** Simmer pears in a mixture of water, cinnamon, and a splash of honey until tender. Top with a generous portion of Greek yogurt.

10.3 Light and Refreshing Options

Sometimes, you want a dessert that's light and refreshing. These options fit the bill perfectly:

1. **Citrus Salad**:** Combine segments of oranges, grapefruits, and blood oranges. Garnish with fresh mint and drizzle with a little honey.

2. **Watermelon Feta Skewers**:** Thread cubes of watermelon and feta cheese onto skewers.

Sprinkle with a bit of balsamic reduction for a sweet and savory treat.

3. **Lemon Sorbet:** Blend fresh lemon juice with a bit of honey and water. Freeze for a tangy and refreshing sorbet.

4. **Berry Ice Pops:** Puree mixed berries with a bit of water and honey. Pour into molds to make frozen pops, for a refreshing treat.

5. **Cucumber Mint Granita:** Blend cucumber with mint leaves and a bit of lime juice. Freeze and scrape with a fork to create a light and icy dessert.

By incorporating these healthy snacking ideas, finger foods for gatherings, dips and spreads, and sweet, fruit-based, and light desserts into your diet, you'll be able to enjoy a variety of flavors and satisfy your cravings while staying true to the DASH diet principles. These recipes and ideas prove that healthy eating can be both delicious and fun, making it easier to stick with your DASH diet journey.

CHAPTER ELEVEN

7-Day Beginner's Meal Plan

Starting the DASH diet can feel overwhelming, but with a solid plan, you can ease into it smoothly. This 7-day beginner's meal plan is designed to help you get acquainted with the DASH diet principles while enjoying a variety of delicious meals.

11.1 Daily Menus

Day 1:

1. **Breakfast:** Greek yogurt with mixed berries and a sprinkle of granola

2. **Lunch:** Quinoa salad with black beans, corn, and avocado

3. **Snack:** Apple slices with almond butter

4. **Dinner:** Baked salmon with steamed broccoli and brown rice

Day 2:

1. **Breakfast:** Oatmeal topped with banana slices and a dash of cinnamon

2. **Lunch:** Turkey and avocado wrap with a side of baby carrots

3. **Snack:** Handful of mixed nuts

4. **Dinner:** Chicken stir-fry with mixed vegetables over brown rice

Day 3:

1. **Breakfast:** Smoothie with spinach, banana, and almond milk

2. **Lunch:** Spinach and strawberry salad with balsamic vinaigrette

3. **Snack:** Greek yogurt with honey and walnuts

4. **Dinner:** Lentil soup with whole grain bread

Day 4:

1. **Breakfast:** Whole grain toast with avocado and a poached egg

2. **Lunch:** Mediterranean chickpea salad

3. **Snack:** Sliced cucumber with hummus

4. **Dinner:** Grilled chicken with roasted sweet potatoes and green beans

Day 5:

1. **Breakfast:** Chia seed pudding topped with fresh mango

2. **Lunch:** Butternut squash soup with a side of mixed greens

3. **Snack:** Orange slices

4. **Dinner:** Shrimp and vegetable skewers with quinoa pilaf

Day 6:

1. **Breakfast:** Berry parfait with Greek yogurt and nuts

2. **Lunch:** Chicken Caesar salad with light dressing

3. **Snack:** Bell pepper strips with guacamole

4. **Dinner:** Stuffed bell peppers with a side of sautéed spinach

Day 7:

1. **Breakfast:** Smoothie with mixed berries, spinach, and coconut water

2. **Lunch:** Tuna salad on whole grain bread with cherry tomatoes

3. **Snack:** Fresh pineapple slices

4. **Dinner:** Baked cod with garlic green beans and cauliflower mash

11.2   Recipes and Prep Tips

Baked Salmon:ll

1. Preheat the oven to 375°F.

2. Place salmon filets on a baking sheet, drizzle with olive oil, and season with lemon juice, dill, salt, and pepper.

3. Bake for 15-20 minutes until flaky.

Quinoa Salad:

1. Cook 1 cup quinoa according to package instructions.

2. Mix cooked quinoa with 1 can of black beans (drained), 1 cup corn, 1 diced red bell pepper, 1 avocado (cubed), and 1/4 cup chopped cilantro.

3. Dress with juice of 1 lime, 2 tbsp olive oil, and 1 tsp cumin.

Lentil Soup:

1. In a large pot, sauté 1 diced onion, 2 chopped carrots, and 2 chopped celery stalks in 2 tbsp olive oil until tender.

2. Add 2 minced garlic cloves and cook for another minute.

3. Add 1 cup lentils, 1 can diced tomatoes, and 4 cups low-sodium vegetable broth.

4. Season with 1 tsp thyme, 1 bay leaf, salt, and pepper.

5. Simmer for 30-40 minutes until the lentils are tender.

CHAPTER TWELVE

14+7-Day Advanced Meal Plan

Once you've mastered the basics of the DASH diet, it's time to dive deeper with a more comprehensive 14+7-day advanced meal plan. This plan will introduce you to a wider variety of meals, offering more complexity and diversity in flavors.

12.1 Comprehensive Guide

Day 1-7:

1. **Day 1:** Whole grain pancakes with blueberries, grilled vegetable and quinoa bowl, bell peppers with tzatziki, baked chicken with walnut crust, roasted Brussels sprouts, and wild rice.

2. **Day 2:** Smoothie bowl with spinach, kiwi, and chia seeds, spicy black bean soup with whole grain crackers, mango slices with chili powder, seared tuna steak with sesame crust, cucumber salad, and soba noodles.

3. **Day 3:** Avocado toast with poached egg and berries, roasted beet and goat cheese salad with walnuts and arugula, Greek yogurt with honey and almonds, vegetable lasagna with whole wheat noodles.

4. **Day 4:** Chia pudding with coconut milk and tropical fruits, stuffed portobello mushrooms with quinoa, spinach, and feta, carrot sticks with almond butter, shrimp and vegetable stir-fry with brown rice and steamed edamame.

5. **Day 5:** Greek yogurt with honey and nuts, lentil and vegetable soup, sliced cucumber with hummus, grilled salmon with quinoa pilaf and asparagus.

6. **Day 6:** Smoothie with mixed berries, kale, and almond milk, turkey and avocado wrap, apple slices with peanut butter, chicken stir-fry with brown rice and mixed vegetables.

7. **Day 7:** Oatmeal with banana and chia seeds, spinach and strawberry salad, Greek yogurt with granola, baked cod with roasted vegetables and wild rice.

Day 8-14: +7

1. **Day 8:** Whole grain toast with avocado and poached egg, butternut squash soup, bell pepper strips with guacamole, grilled chicken with sweet potato and green beans.

2. **Day 9:** Chia seed pudding with mango, tuna salad on whole grain bread, carrot sticks with almond butter, shrimp skewers with quinoa and vegetable medley.

3. **Day 10:** Smoothie bowl with mixed berries and chia seeds, roasted beet salad with walnuts, Greek yogurt with honey and almonds, vegetable lasagna with whole wheat noodles.

4. **Day 11:** Avocado toast with poached egg and berries, quinoa salad with black beans, apple slices with peanut butter, chicken stir-fry with brown rice and mixed vegetables.

5. **Day 12:** Greek yogurt with berries and nuts, Mediterranean chickpea salad, cucumber slices with hummus, grilled salmon with quinoa pilaf and asparagus.

6. **Day 13:** Oatmeal with banana and chia seeds, spinach and strawberry salad, bell pepper strips with guacamole, baked cod with roasted vegetables and wild rice.

7. **Day 14:** Smoothie with spinach, banana, and almond milk, turkey and avocado wrap, sliced cucumber with hummus, shrimp and vegetable stir-fry with brown rice and steamed edamame.

12.2 Recipes and Shopping Lists

Whole Grain Pancakes:

1. Mix 1 cup whole grain flour, 1 tbsp baking powder, 1/2 tsp salt, 1 cup almond milk, 1 egg, and 2 tbsp olive oil.
- Heat the griddle until bubbles appear on the surface, then turn and continue cooking until the food turns golden brown.

Grilled Vegetable and Quinoa Bowl:

1. Grill a mix of zucchini, bell peppers, eggplant, and asparagus.

2. Serve over cooked quinoa, drizzled with a tahini dressing (2 tbsp tahini, juice of 1 lemon, 1 tbsp olive oil, 1 minced garlic clove, and water to thin).

Seared Tuna Steak:

1. Coat tuna steak in sesame seeds.

2. Sear in a hot pan with a little olive oil for about 2 minutes on each side for medium-rare.

Shopping List:

1. Whole grain flour, almond milk, eggs, Greek yogurt, quinoa, a variety of fresh vegetables, lean meats, nuts, seeds, low-sodium broth, whole wheat pasta, and fresh fruits.

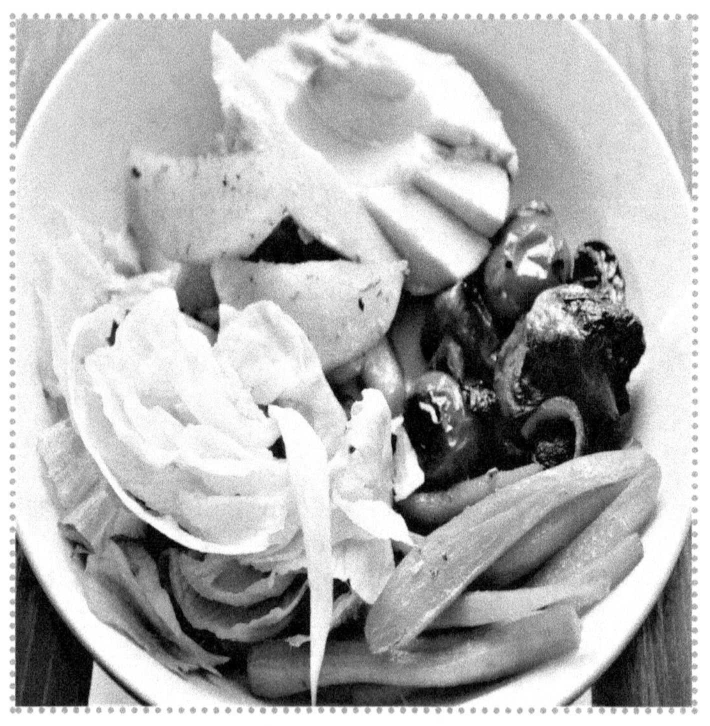

CHAPTER THIRTEEN

Tips and Strategies for Success

Maintaining a healthy diet can be challenging, especially when dining out or during social events. This chapter offers practical tips and strategies to help you make healthy choices on the DASH diet, no matter the situation.

13.1 Eating Out on the DASH Diet

Your good eating habits don't have to be destroyed by eating out. The following advice will help you stay focused:

1. **Plan Ahead:** Check the restaurant's menu online before you go and choose dishes that align with the DASH diet.

2. **Ask for Modifications:** Don't hesitate to ask for changes, such as dressing on the side, grilled instead of fried, or extra vegetables instead of starch.

3. **Portion Control:** Restaurant portions are often large. Consider sharing a dish or asking for a to-go box at the start of the meal to pack half away.

13.2   Making Healthy Choices at Restaurants

When dining out, these strategies can help you make healthier choices:

1. **Opt for Lean Proteins:** Choose dishes that feature chicken, fish, or plant-based proteins.

2. **Load Up on Veggies:** Look for meals that include a generous portion of vegetables, or order a side of steamed veggies or a salad.

3. **Watch the Sodium:** Ask for low-sodium options or request that no additional salt be added to your meal.

13.3   Tips for Social Events and Holidays

Social events and holidays can be particularly challenging, but with a little planning, you can enjoy these occasions while sticking to your DASH diet:

1. **Bring a Healthy Dish**:** If you're attending a potluck or family gathering, bring a dish that you know aligns with your dietary goals.

2. **Stay Hydrated**:** Drink plenty of water, which can help you feel full and avoid overeating

.

3. **Mindful Eating**:** Pay attention to the company and food you are enjoying. Eat mindfully, slowly, and enjoy every bite while gauging your level of hunger and fullness.

4. **Balance Indulgences**:** It's okay to enjoy special treats, but try to balance them with healthier options and keep portion sizes in check.

By following these tips and strategies, you can navigate eating out, social events, and holidays while staying committed to your DASH diet goals. Remember, flexibility and balance are key to long-term success and

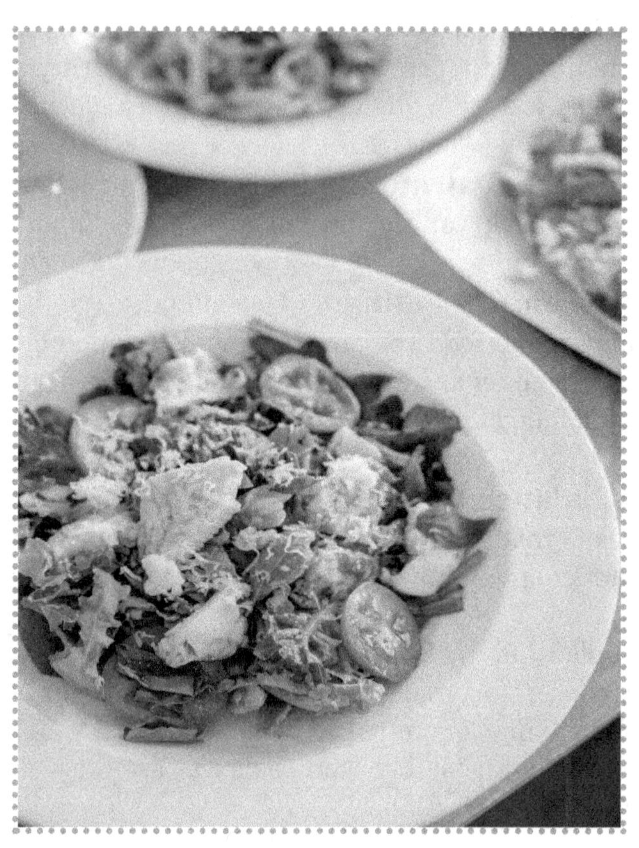

CHAPTER FOURTEEN

Staying Motivated and On Track

Sticking to a new diet can be challenging, but staying motivated and tracking your progress can make a significant difference. Here are some strategies to help you stay on course with the DASH diet.

14.1   Setting Realistic Goals

Establishing attainable and reasonable goals is essential for long-term success. Instead of aiming for drastic changes, focus on small, manageable steps.

1. **Start Small:** Begin with simple goals, like reducing your soda intake or incorporating more vegetables into your meals.

2. **Be Specific:** Rather than a vague goal like "eat healthier," set specific targets like "eat five servings of fruits and vegetables daily."

3. **Trackable Goals:** Ensure your goals are measurable. For example, "exercise for 30 minutes, three times a week" is a clear, trackable goal.

14.2   Tracking Your Progress

Keeping track of your progress helps you stay motivated and see the improvements you're making.

1. **Food Diary:** Maintain a food diary to record what you eat and drink. You can use this to spot trends and make the required corrections.

2. **Regular Weigh-Ins:** Weigh yourself regularly but not obsessively. Weekly check-ins can give you a sense of your progress without causing undue stress.

3. 3. **Honor Milestones:** Honor your accomplishments, no matter how modest. Rewarding yourself for meeting your goals can boost motivation.

14.3   Overcoming Common Challenges

Everyone faces obstacles when trying to stick to a new diet. Here are some tips to overcome common challenges:

1. **Busy Schedules:** Plan and prepare meals ahead of time. You can save time throughout the week by doing bulk cooking on the weekends.

2. **Social Pressures:** Communicate your dietary goals to friends and family. They can offer support and may even join you in making healthier choices.

3. **Cravings:** Find healthier alternatives to your favorite treats. If you crave something sweet, try fruit-based desserts or dark chocolate in moderation.

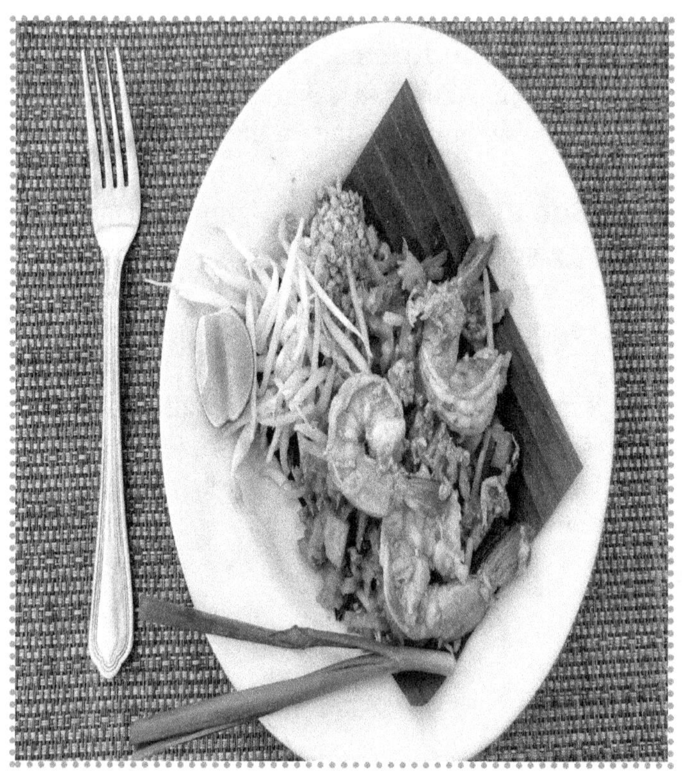

CHAPTER FIFTEEN

CONCLUSION

As you reach the end of this cookbook, it's time to reflect on your journey and look ahead to your continued success on the DASH diet.

15.1 Your Journey to Better Health

Embarking on the DASH diet is a step towards better health and well-being. By choosing nutritious, balanced meals, you're not only improving your physical health but also enhancing your quality of life.

1. **Reflect on Your Progress:** Take a moment to acknowledge how far you've come. Reflect on the positive changes in your diet, energy levels, and overall health.

2. **Learn from Experience:** Identify what strategies worked best for you and what areas might need adjustment. Apply these learnings to future iterations of your strategy.

15.2   Continuing Your DASH Diet Journey

Sticking with the DASH diet is a lifelong commitment to healthier eating habits. Here's how to maintain your progress:

1. **Stay Educated:** Continue learning about nutrition and exploring new recipes. This will keep your meals engaging and help you avoid getting bored.

2. **Adapt and Adjust:** Your dietary needs may change over time. Be flexible and willing to adjust your diet as needed.

3. **Seek Support:** Surround yourself with supportive friends, family, or online communities. Having other people witness your path can help to hold you accountable and encourage you.

15.3   Additional Resources and Support

Utilize additional resources to stay informed and motivated:

1.   **Books and Websites**:** Explore books and websites dedicated to the DASH diet for new recipes and tips.

2.   **Apps**:** Use mobile apps for meal planning, grocery shopping, and tracking your progress

.

3.   **Professional Support**:** Consider consulting a dietitian or nutritionist for personalized advice and support.

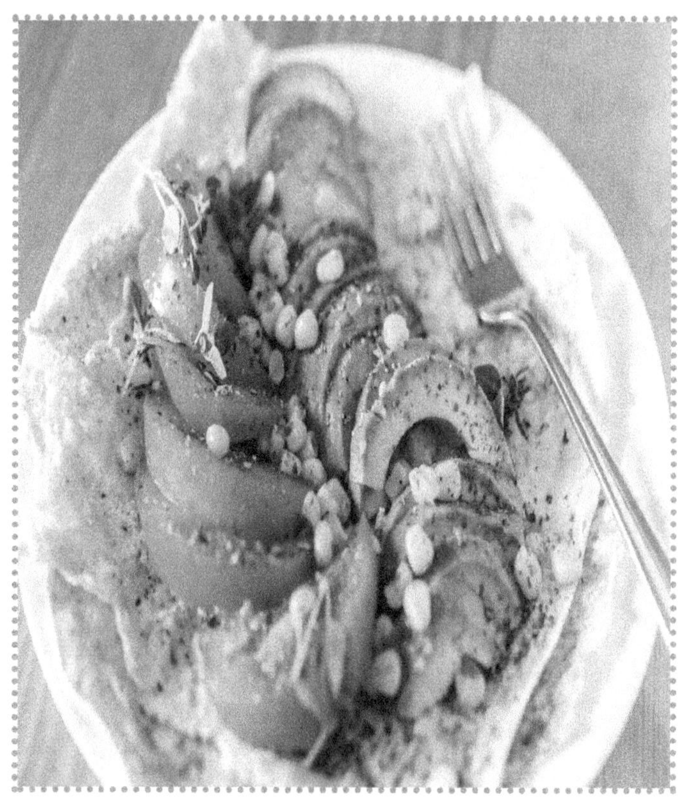

CHAPTER SIXTEEN

Appendices

Appendix A:

DASH Diet Food Lists

Having a comprehensive list of approved foods can make it easier to plan your meals and ensure you're following the DASH diet correctly. Here's a detailed list to guide you.

1. **Fruits:** Apples, bananas, berries, citrus fruits, melons, peaches, pears

2. **Vegetables:** Leafy greens (spinach, kale), broccoli, carrots, tomatoes, bell peppers, squash

3. **Whole Grains:** Whole wheat bread, brown rice, quinoa, oatmeal, whole grain pasta

4. **Lean Proteins:** Chicken breast, turkey, fish, tofu, legumes (beans, lentils), nuts, and seeds

5. **Dairy:** Low-fat or fat-free milk, yogurt, cheese

6. **Healthy Fats:** Olive oil, avocado, nuts, and seeds

7 **Beverages:** Water, herbal teas, limited amounts of 100% fruit juice

16.2   Comprehensive List of Approved Foods

This list provides a quick reference to ensure you're incorporating a variety of foods that align with the DASH diet principles.

1. **Proteins:** Skinless poultry, lean beef, pork tenderloin, seafood, eggs, plant-based proteins (beans, peas, lentils)

2. **Grains:** Whole wheat products, bulgur, barley, farro, millet, whole corn

3. **Dairy:** Skim or 1% milk, low-fat cheese, Greek yogurt, cottage cheese

4. **Vegetables:** Asparagus, Brussels sprouts, cauliflower, cucumbers, eggplant, mushrooms

5. **Fruits:** Grapes, kiwi, mango, pineapple, watermelon

6. **Nuts and Seeds:** Almonds, walnuts, sunflower seeds, chia seeds, flaxseeds

7. **Healthy Fats:** Canola oil, sunflower oil, nut butters

By following these food lists and incorporating the tips and strategies outlined in this cookbook, you'll be well-equipped to succeed on your DASH diet journey. Remember, the key is consistency and making informed choices that contribute to your overall health and well-being.